SATISFYING HIM IN BED

How To Please Your Man Sexually And Make Him Climb The Wall Of Ecstasy

Helen D. Seaman

FOR MY MAN

TABLE OF CONTENTS

"Making you aroused and making you smile are my two favorite things."

"TLDR; let go of the pressure, focus on the pleasure."

Introduction

Become a knowledgeable lover to greatly improve your sex life.

Let's have an open dialogue. Sex is wonderful and essential to a happy relationship. Along with being wild, entertaining, exciting, and exhilarating, it also leaves you with a tremendous yearning. Additionally, it fosters a deeper spiritual and emotional bond between you and your particular someone.

Even while sex is wonderful, there are some aspects of it that can be unpleasant. To mention a few, your spouse might not make you happy, certain situations might be a little uncomfortable, there might be something lacking between the two of you, or you might both be performing roles that you don't particularly enjoy.

It's crucial to remember that it's normal to have favorite and least favorite sex positions. Furthermore, it's critical to keep in mind that different sex positions appeal to different people in different ways. Even when it comes to sex, everyone has various preferences and desires.

CHAPTER 1 - How to Arouse a Man!

Sometimes you have to be inventive and venture into the forbidden territory to arouse your man.

Now, doesn't that sound alluring? But it's accurate.

Women are desperate to learn more about what they can do to make their man content, if not thrilled.

Ah, but the question of how to promote arousal is not really a straightforward one.

Additionally, arousal isn't always brought on by what a woman does for her husband or boyfriend. When we discuss the relationship arousal equation, there is a lot more to it.

When a woman knows her man is highly stimulated, she feels stimulated, and vice versa. Keep this in mind. This subject will be covered again later.

But let's move on to your man's most basic aspirations. If you are willing to experiment with new sexual encounters (with each other) and experiences, it can be very stimulating for both the husband and wife.

A man occasionally considers engaging in sexual activity with his wife that might push them close to the Forbidden Zone. Even just him thinking about such things can arouse. It's like a summons to his "primal" self, where he imagines a sensual encounter that is unrefined, sweaty, wild, and exhilarating.

Of course, it doesn't have to be quite that way, but your man likes to think in those terms. You can make use of those ideas.

Additionally, he may find it very exciting if he thinks that you may be considering exploring the "forbidden zone" as well.

Keeping things vague is crucial. Less can be more.

Give your husband (or boyfriend) the freedom to use his own imagination to try to fill in the blanks. You can create a masterpiece of arousal if you are very cunning and just a little bit sinister.

You could, for instance, send him a cryptic text message an hour before he gets home from work.

Alternately, you could hide an envelope for him to find later.

Let it all take in and gradually develop. This is how arousal manifests in your man. It begins as a fleeting thought in the mind.

What Other Initiatives Can You Undertake To Accomplish Arousal?

For men, certain colors can be very seductive. For instance, wearing red can signal your readiness, which makes your husband or boyfriend more aroused.

However, our discussion will go beyond how colors affect a man's mood. If you must know, "black" also functions.

Let's move forward.

I enjoy coming up with novel ways to pose the same query. If we don't push ourselves to broaden our knowledge and experiences, we can frequently become fixed in one way of doing things. Sometimes, simply asking the question repeatedly can lead to the discovery of original and inventive solutions.

However, I'm not done with you yet! Let's discuss some of the supporting science that relates to this topic before you leave.

What else do you need to understand about sexual intimacy and arousal in order to be a better wife and companion to your husband (or boyfriend)?

Let's discuss Oxytocin.

The better your understanding of this hormone, the more.

It functions as both a neurotransmitter and a hormone. This fantastic chemical is released by your pituitary gland. However, let me give you a quick crash course in Oxytocin just in case you forgot! The hormone oxytocin, which is released by the brain, is considered to be a crucial chemical messenger for influencing human behavior. It contributes to arousing us to the point where we can feel turned on by the smallest touches or glances.

You came here specifically to learn more about that, after all. A chemical reaction can occur in the brain even in response to the smallest touches or stray glances.

Oxytocin promotes sexual arousal.

This wonderful hormone of love aids our ability to perceive reality. It improves our capacity for clearer perception and experience. Because of the impact it has on us, we can learn to trust and confide even our most intimate secrets. We are able to develop the strongest of attachments because of the release of oxytocin in our brains (bonding). Additionally, oxytocin is known to ease tension and encourage sleep. It resembles a miracle drug. Finding a way to naturally produce it is difficult because, once it is released into our brain chemistry, we experience an unparalleled high. I suppose that's why it's known as the "love hormone" or the "cuddle chemical" by so many people.

You must admit that it sounds fairly good. However, I believe I understand your thoughts as well! How do I get this juice flowing in my head and in my husband's or boyfriend's head? is probably what you're wondering.

A good query. We can't hand it out like candy, though. We also can't use it to make a batch of cookies.

It is formed as a result of triggers. What then are these catalysts that increase oxytocin? If I were you, I'm sure I would be thinking the same thing.

Let's discuss that, then. Here are some actions you can take with and around your partner that have been shown to act as oxytocin release triggers.

- Hugging
- Laughter and a smile
- Long-lasting eye contact
- Making eye contact and grinning together can be highly effective.
- For ladies: Wearing a stylish red dress or attire communicates readiness for sexual activity
- For males: Red clothing conveys strength and better status.
- Touching very lightly and subtly
- Walking quickly and exercising (endorphins are released)
- Playing nice music
- Singing
- Communicating private information
- Showing goodwill

- Use a voice with a deeper pitch (men)
- Use a higher-pitched voice, but not one that is too high (women)
- Displaying your neck's curve, a limp wrist, and large lips outward (women)
- Provoking your man to sex
- Leaning in and showing your boyfriend some compassion
- Mirroring (when you replicate your husband motions and actions)

When it comes to enticing your lover, talking is overrated!

I know! I know! It nearly has a blasphemous tone. Pick up lines, in fact, are an entire industry unto themselves. But did you know that only 7% of communication—the majority of which happens nonverbally—leads to attraction? Therefore, your man is not clinging to words.

In essence, research has shown that talking is not as important as thought.

The majority of the pick up lines we hear about fail. The nonverbal forms of communication rule the day when you start dissecting and finding all of the ways in which we communicate and aligning them with what attracts.

How does that appear numerically then? It turns out that our vocal tones make up about 45% and our body language, such as our posture and facial expressions, makes up about 60%.

It's crucial to understand that this numerical breakdown holds true when people discuss their feelings and levels of attraction for one another. It appears that non-verbal indications from a person are more perceptible to us. The fact that people tend to make up their minds about what they find beautiful rather rapidly is another intriguing fact.

You typically become turned on by something practically instantaneously. Additionally, figuring out if you are attracted to someone does not take very long. It is stated that after the conversation begins, a person will often know if they are attracted to another between 90 seconds to 4 minutes.

As a result, as you can see, this emphasizes the importance of the first minutes of anything you intend to say in order to maximize attraction levels.

Looking into your husband's eyes can arouse him.

Therefore, if you want to arouse your boyfriend, think about looking into his eyes intently while discussing something incredibly private.

Your man is probably the type of guy that takes action first!

Although nonverbal cues appear to be the main draw, I tend to think more practically. There is always conversation going on. However, there are obvious distinctions between how men and women speak in general. Understanding these differences will benefit you.

Women typically chat to one another to establish a connection.

If you examine how boys and girls interact on a playground, you will see that girls tend to pair off more often and start conversations with one another in order to build connections.

The lads will be playing rough and tumble games while racing around. The boys will frequently instigate hostile, competitive situations.

While the females may be engaged in activities, they are typically having more private conversations and forging friendly social connections.

Even when boys grow up to become men, some aspects of our nature remain relatively unchanged. As we age, certain of our preferences do not become more refined. Men aren't generally regarded as being as social as women in various situations. They frequently withdraw inside of themselves. We frequently choose to withdraw inside our man cave to unwind in order to later come out firing.

Inform your man that listening to you makes you feel seductive.

For wanting to talk little, guys are frequently criticized.

If your man starts to lose interest in what you have to say, don't be too shocked. It's just the way men are wired, in many ways. Your guy likes to be on the go, pursuing opportunities, taking on challenges, and fixing issues. It reminds me a lot of the time when men tracked, hunted, and fought to survive. Women frequently discuss their issues in order to find potential solutions. Men often bottle them up and internalize the problem.

An individual retreats to his cave. A woman is more open-minded and favors honest and productive discussion of the relationship. Most men have relatively short attention spans. They enjoy figuring out problems. They have been programmed in this way.

Your husband is programmed to look for a solution if he hears you talking about a problem you are having. Your husband will feel more confident and prepared to tackle the next challenge or activity on his to-do list after offering solutions to your problem.

But here is the catch. The majority of men fail to realize that you will feel safe, supported, and loved if he takes the time to slow down and simply listen to you. Therefore, express to him how listening to you makes you feel a certain way.

When their husband or boyfriend really listens to them, many women have told me, it literally turns them on. In some cases, it already is. Sometimes it happens later. However, the bond and connection they have with their boyfriend (or husband) at that precise moment is obvious.

I have heard time and time again that the best sex that women have experienced with their husbands (or boyfriends) often occurs after he patiently listens to what she has to say and offers support.

The Major Disconnection That Extinguishes Arousal

The best and the worst things about relationships are communication between the sexes.

Although there is a wide range of possibilities, I want every couple I work with to recognize that communication in a relationship is inherently flawed. It needs to be improved. Understanding the distinctions between men and women's communication preferences is helpful for moving forward.

Keep in mind that, in our subconscious, men are hunters and protectors. They frequently desire to go back to our cave or spend time with our male buddies when we need some downtime.

So allow him.

Women are typically considerably more perceptive and adept at doing so. They are able to process information in various dimensions.

Men prefer to receive things one at a time. They typically struggle to understand their wife's (or girlfriend's) thoughts. Get ready to be let down if you recently got a little different hairstyle and are teasing your guy about it. He was most likely unaware of the distinction.

Therefore, don't blame him.

The language that men employ is typically more direct. When they inquire, "How's it going?" You then say, "I guess it's alright." A guy would assume everything was good.

He rarely makes inquiries or establishes lines of connection. A woman, on the other hand, will explore and broaden the discourse since she has a tendency to understand the underlying intricacy of social language.

In order to gently encourage him to probe more in the future, start by complimenting him. Most men prefer to be active. They are focused on the body. When they are active, they feel better, think better, and process better.

So, if a woman wants a guy to talk openly, seize the chance to work out with him. Workout with him.

I'll let you in on a little secret, though.

You must broaden your understanding of effective communication if you want to maximize "attraction" and get your man "all worked up." Intimacy and arousal have little room to grow when disagreements and poor communication get in the way.

Educate Your Man On How To Make You Excited

Teach your husband or boyfriend how to get you excited if you really want to get a rise out of him. His nonconscious sensor will detect those signals when you are activated, which will thrill him.

It seems like a win-win situation to me.

The majority of men have no idea how to approach a woman romantically. Most men need instruction on what it is that makes you excited. It might be a chore for some guys to follow instructions. The "Casanova Syndrome" affects a lot of guys, making them believe that everything they say and do is flawless.

How do you solve this issue?

Although it might sound radical, I would advise you to discuss the things you and your partner enjoy doing.

Although talking about such things is hardly novel, you might be surprised at how rarely such conversations occur. But it's well known that there are differences between men and women in their comprehension of the subtler aspects of attraction.

You must therefore discuss your shared likes and dislikes. But before we get into that, let's talk about some universal principles that hold true for both men and women.

What Stirs a Woman Up?

Keep in mind that in order to convey the unconscious signals that your man's brain interprets as "sex," you must be genuinely excited.

This section of this book is sort of dedicated to your husband. However, you may train him. Women frequently like slow romance. Little things add up. Less is more is a great mantra to use as a guideline for your love correspondence.

Your man must be aware of this.

This whole idea of the gradual romance could appear completely backwards to your husband. Your hubby moves much more quickly by nature. But your man genuinely wants to win your favor. Encourage him to take things slowly because doing so will make him really happy.

You should discuss active listening with your husband.

Your lover may initially think it's a foreign language, but eventually he'll realize that eye contact-heavy listening is the surest path to winning your heart.

Remind him of how much you appreciate him staring into your eyes. Tell him you enjoy it. He will become agitated by that blunt language.

Remember that when lovers look into each other's eyes, the brain is predisposed to release oxytocin, which causes desire.

When you use the proper body language, there is a beautiful synergy between you and your boyfriend.

Keep in mind to physically lean into conversations with your husband. Thank your man for his sincere interest in what you have to say.

Men enjoy being stroked. Unknown to him, your husband's ego is a priceless asset.

Lean in and make the most of it by boosting his ego. Examine his eyes. He'll feel more in control, and you look stunning in that picture.

I would tell your husband or significant other if they were present.

How Can You Make Your Man More Intimate?

Unfortunately, I can't guarantee that your man is eagerly awaiting each word I type right now!

Let's discuss how to improve your relationship with your partner so that he is more available to you. Oddly, there are times when you need to give him space if you want his full focus or, more specifically, if you want to get him a little sexy.

What then can you say to a guy to get their heart to open up and increase intimacy?

You must first realize that men think about things differently than women. The majority of the time, your boyfriend (or husband) struggles with sharing. Men dislike being confined. We desire a sense of authority and control. We would rather engage in sexual activity before speaking. We are quick to act and strong defenders.

So how do you deal with a guy's preferences for intimacy and communication?

You see, some men struggle with attachment. They value their freedom and do not want to be possessed. Our insecurities may be caused by these things. Your guy will open up after you remove that worry.

Hearing this kind of language is really attractive to men. They want to "own" you during the act of sexual closeness, even though they don't want to entirely give themselves up (in some aspects). It appeals to their emotional monster.

Numerous intriguing hormones can be released during sex, which promotes intimacy and closeness.

Therefore, you can utilize what I refer to as "Turn On" language with a twist if you want to find out what your guy is truly thinking about the relationship.

A man's instinct is to defend. When you tell them that, it makes your man feel powerful and important. But be careful not to overdo it; keep it brief so a guy won't perceive you as being overly dependent. Men can experience body insecurity, just like women do. Don't gush over his appearance. Just a quick comment, please. It will boost his ego and make him appear more approachable and sexually attractive.

Happy romantic endeavors until then.

CHAPTER 2 - Beliefs about male sex drive

Men are frequently portrayed as sex-obsessed machines in stereotypes. Characters and plot points in books, television shows, and films frequently presuppose that men are obsessive sex addicts and women are only interested in romance.

Is it real, though? What do we know about a man's desire for sex?

Prejudices against men's sex drive

What myths about a man's sex drive are thus true? How do men stack up against women? Let's examine these prevalent misconceptions about male sexuality.

Men consider having sex all day.

The common misconception that men think about sex every seven seconds has been disproved by a recent study at Ohio State University involving over 200 students. That translates to 8,000 thoughts in 16 hours of awake time. The study's young men reported having sex thoughts 19 times on average daily. The study's young participants said they had 10 thoughts about sex on average each day.

So, do men consider sex twice as often as women do? The study also suggested that men had more frequent thoughts about eating and sleeping than did women. It's possible that men feel more at ease reporting their thoughts on sex than women do.

Men engage in masturbation more frequently than women.

In a 2009 study on 600 adults in Guangzhou, China, 48.8% of female participants and 68.7% of male participants admitted to masturbating. The survey also indicated that a sizable portion of adults, particularly women, had a negative opinion of masturbation.

Men are more amenable to casual sex than women.

According to a 2015 study, men are more likely than women to partake in casual sex. In the study, 162 men and 119 women were approached at a nightclub or on a college campus by 6 men and 8 women. They sent out a request for light sexual activity. Men took up the offer at a significantly higher rate than women did.

But in the second phase of the same study, these researchers found that women seemed more receptive to invitations for casual sex when they were in a secure setting. Women and men were shown images of potential suitors and questioned about their willingness to engage in casual sex. When women thought they were in a safer environment, the gender gap in responses vanished.

The discrepancy between these two studies suggests that social norms and other cultural factors can significantly influence how men and women look for intimate partners.

Men are not as romantic as women are.

People's sources of arousal can differ greatly from one another. The way that men and women experience sexuality and how they report it in surveys are frequently shaped by sexual norms and taboos. Because of this, it is challenging to demonstrate scientifically that men lack a biological propensity for romantic arousal.

The brain and sexual desire

Libido is frequently used to indicate sex urge. Libido cannot be measured numerically. Instead, sex drive is defined in ways that are pertinent. For instance, a reduced libido translates into a diminished interest in or desire for sex.

The limbic system and the cerebral cortex are where the male libido resides in the brain. These brain regions are essential to a man's sex drive and functionality. In fact, they are so crucial that a man can have an orgasm just by daydreaming or thinking about a sexual encounter.

The gray matter that makes up the brain's outer layer is known as the cerebral cortex. It is the area of your brain that is in charge of higher-level operations like thinking and planning. This includes having sex in mind. Signals from the cerebral cortex can interact with other areas of the brain and nerves when you become aroused. Some of these nerves increase blood supply to your genitalia and pulse rate. They also signal the erection-producing process.

The hippocampus, hypothalamus, amygdala, and other brain regions are included in the limbic system. These areas are connected to emotion, drive, and sex desire.

Testosterone

The hormone most closely linked to male sex drive is testosterone. Testosterone, which is primarily produced in the testicles, is essential for a variety of bodily processes, including:

- Creation of male genitalia
- Body hair, bone, and muscular mass increase, and the voice becomes deeper throughout puberty.
- Sperm generation
- Red blood cell formation
- Red blood cell formation

A decreased libido is frequently associated with low testosterone levels. In general, testosterone levels rise in the morning and fall at night. A man's lifetime testosterone levels peak in his late teens, and then they gradually start to fall.

Loss of libido

Age might cause a decline in sex desire. However, there are situations when a libido decline is related to a more serious issue. Reduced sex drive can result from the following factors:

Depression or stress. Speak with your doctor if you are suffering mental health problems. He or she might propose treatment or provide a prescription for medicine.

Endocrine problems. Male sex hormone levels could drop due to an endocrine condition.

Low levels of testosterone. Low testosterone levels, which can have an effect on your sex desire, can be brought on by certain medical problems like sleep apnea.

Certain medicines. Your libido may be impacted by several drugs. A few antidepressants, antihistamines, and even blood pressure drugs, for example, might make erections difficult. Your doctor might be able to offer a substitute.

Elevated blood pressure. A man's capacity to achieve or maintain an erection might be negatively impacted by vascular system damage.

Diabetes. Diabetes, like high blood pressure, can harm a man's vascular system and impair his capacity to keep an erection for long periods of time.

The only person who can gauge how normal your sex drive is you. Consult your doctor if you notice changes in your libido. Even though it can be challenging at times, a medical expert could be able to assist you talk to someone about your sexual preferences.

Outlook

Does a man's sex drive ever stop? For many men, the libido never truly goes away. Libido will most likely fluctuate over time for most men. It's possible that with time, both the frequency and the method you enjoy sex will alter. However, having sex and being intimate can be enjoyable as we age.

CHAPTER 3 - Seducing a man in front of others

The ability to seduce your man is more seductive than anything else. Have you ever wondered what other carefully thought-out actions you might be able to take to make him want more if just one flick of your hair does it? You'll become completely irresistible in his eyes by using the next 20 seduction strategies.

1. Open the show.

It's best to take the lead in the bedroom. Men like identifying "bad girl" traits in their girlfriends. Take his hand and lead him into the bedroom. Or, if he frequently assumes this role, make the request for him to go with you home yourself. Who knows, perhaps a slight role-reversal will show you in a new light!

2. *Belittle him*

It's common knowledge that most men like to be teased! Come up to him, kiss him on the mouth, and walk away. Several times, repeat this. Make him hanker after you. But keep things lighthearted so he won't be confused by what's happening.

3. *Allow him to see an anecdote.*

Wear something that gives him a hint of what he might be getting to play with later that night, but don't go overboard. Simple things like leaving the extra button on your shirt undone work. Wearing nothing but a plain white t-shirt, try joining him in the shower. The best sneak peek imaginable is that one!

4. Present food.

Really, it doesn't have to be a complete mess. Simply lick your fingers clean after removing the whipped cream from your coffee, or take a more enticing bite out of your strawberry. That almost always yields breathtaking outcomes!

5. Go commando to ensure he is aware.

The next moment you go out to dinner, skip the underwear and tell him in a quiet voice while you're still eating. After that, we can guarantee that all of his attention will be focused on getting you alone.

6. Put on blinders.

If you're not afraid to try something new, put a blindfold on him. Alternatively, use your handkerchief or his tie. Then take his hands and wrap them around your waist before giving him a long, passionate kiss.

7. Curl your lower lip.

Your verbal communication has a big influence on what he is thinking. For instance, if you lightly bite your bottom while you two are conversing, he might not notice, but that little act will stay in his mind all night long!

8. Always have a great scent

A man finds nothing more alluring than a woman with a particularly alluring scent. Don't go overboard, though. With just a few strategically placed sprays of your best cologne, he ought to be able to smell it (from a little distance away).

9. Set the mood with some music.

Of course, the environment is important! Play some sensual but romantic music and start it as soon as he enters the room. Ask him to join you as you dance a little bit. After all, one of the sexiest forms of foreplay in the world is dance!

10. Shapen your cleavage.

Girls, put your knowledge of makeup to use. Accentuate and contour your cleavage for best results! With this little effort, you'll undoubtedly get some of the extra attention you deserve!

11. Put the "No Hands Rule" to use.

The secret to a great relationship with your partner is spontaneity. Why don't you try the "No Hands Rule" then? Before you start kissing him, make it clear that he is not permitted to touch you. He won't be able to hold out against you for long, we guarantee it!

12. Increase Excitement with Text

Even though bedroom tricks are great on their own, it's a good idea to use text messages to build anticipation for what will happen.

A man can be seduced very successfully by texting. How? He will be eager to meet you as soon as you text him a list of everything he can look forward to that evening.

13. *Go shopping with him!*

No, we're not talking about the typical shopping trip that you'd probably prefer not to take your partner on. When we ask you to bring him along, we're talking about going lingerie shopping. The excitement will increase once you inquire as to what he hopes to see you wearing.

14. *Surprise Him!*

Surprise always gives a bedtime activity a little extra spice. If you've been dating for some time, this might work especially well since he's probably used to seeing you in your faithful pajamas and a messy bun. Give him a surprise the next time he stops by to see you. To appear as though you are making an effort just for him, dress seductively, put on some makeup, and let your hair down. Surely he'll get involved in this!

15. Have a shower together

This cute little ploy now works best when he least expects it. So, sneak into the bathroom and surprise him when he's alone in the shower. You two are going to get irate over this, I can tell!

16. Invite him for a massage

Even though he might not have asked for a massage directly, you can be sure that he would appreciate it if you acted as his personal masseuse. Then, while he is lying on the bed, give him a thorough massage. As you add some oils to the scene, be sure to touch his delicate areas. Give him a few quick kisses here and there to start things off as a bonus.

17. Participate in a little roleplaying

Believe us when we say that men occasionally enjoy playing role-playing games. So don the attire of his preferred female character and astound him with an outstanding acting display (complete with costumes and everything). Girls, practice your acting skills and prepare to woo him!

18. Play Strip Poker

This one is for long-term relationships where both parties are totally comfortable with one another. If you don't know the rules, the loser of each deal has to take something off. Make sure to lose the game before you start winning it, then! *wink*

19. Engage Him in Public Conversation

For some reason, performing "the act" in public makes it dangerous and seductively intoxicating. Now, we're not suggesting that you go all out for him, but there are unquestionably a lot more subdued options available to you. You could try grazing his leg with your bare feet or lightly touching him underneath the table. These subtle hints, if you understand what we mean, will be sufficient to make him eager for the two of you to return home and be by yourselves.

20. Bring In Some Goodies

It never hurts to try new things if the two of you are comfortable with one another. To add some spontaneity to your sexual life, introduce some goodies. We're discussing sex games that you two can engage in while wearing handcuffs, blindfolds, and other accessories. We're certain that the mere idea would catch his attention.

Now that you know how to woo your guy, what are you waiting for?

CHAPTER 4 - How To Be Irresistible In Bed

It's true what they say: one of the most crucial aspects of a relationship is intimacy. Nobody, however, wants a partner who is uninteresting. We all desire a partner who understands our preferences, points of attraction, and things that make us happy, glowing, and all smiley; the ability to make a man sob in bed can only fuel these sparks.

Wake up from your slumber and adopt these hilariously practical actions if you want to give your man the toe-curling, body-shaking, and mind-blowing sensation that will ultimately make him addicted to you and deepen your relationship.

1. Practice Good Hygiene

The first piece of advice on how to make a man sob in bed tells us to practice good personal hygiene. Take a shower now to ensure that every part of your body is kept clean and appealing.

Wash your lady parts (preferably with water or other safe feminine hygiene products) as you take a shower or bath, paying special attention to the more delicate areas like the ears, neck, armpit, etc.

Use fresh towels, an enticing body lotion, let your hair smell good, polish your fingernails, spritz on a sweet-smelling perfume, and dress to impress.

If you know how to clean up, your man will be charmed every time you are around him. A surefire way to make yourself irresistible to your husband is to keep your home clean.

2. Establish A Mood

Setting a romantic ambiance can only help to increase excitement before we get on the act because it is well known that our environment has an impact on our realities and how we feel.

So make sure your space is welcoming, warm, and well-kept. Purchase sheets (soft, inviting, and snugly fitting on the mattress would do).

If you can, find soft lighting with different light levels for your bedroom. If you can't dim the lights with a dimmer or other device, rewire the lighting so that it uses a nice lamp with a low-wattage bulb instead. Unable to accomplish that

As they soften sharp images and cast a radiant glow all around, scented candles can enhance a sensual mood even further. Additionally, make sure to look amazing in the nastiest piece of underwear you own (it's a tried-and-true method for keeping your man content in bed).

Why not make him fall in love with you all over again by wearing your favorite high heels and sultry red lipstick for the ultimate amazing goddess appeal that he won't be able to resist? With some calming music playing in the background, crawl on all fours towards your romantic lover.

3. Tease a man to make him want you in bed

This is a key component of knowing how to make a man swoon in bed, be irresistible, and make him yearn for you.

When we refer to someone as a tease, we mean that they pretend to give you something that you want but ultimately do not.

To tease your man, get to work! He will be amused if you lean over and playfully pick something up in your short skirt while bending forward to show him your cleavage.

Keep his heart pounding as you carefully and slowly eat that sausage or banana, or draw attention to your mouth with a lollipop in a seductive manner.

If his c*ck were that lollipops, your boyfriend won't be able to stop thinking about what you could have done with your mouth.

You could also eat your food while making out with it. Simply tempt him until he can take it no longer, then watch him unfurl the animalistic passion that even he wasn't aware he possessed as you bite into that fruit and let the juices ooze and drip down your chin.

One of the things your man wants but may be too shy to ask for is to be teased. Get off your high horse and show him your playful side because they usually assume that you know they want you to tease them.

4. Give An Aroused Massage

If you want to know how to make a man cry in bed, don't underestimate the power of a good, deep, and sensual massage. It's one of the routines I've developed in my bedroom over time.

To accomplish this, have your man lie down on the bed while you apply warm oil to his sore body. A sensual head massage can be a great place to start because the scalp contains many stimulating areas. Use slow, circular motions to caress his head to really get him in the mood.

As you approach his face, gently press into his temples with two fingers from each hand for several seconds at a time. You can also use your index finger to trace a soft circle around his lips.

Slowly slide your hands down to his neck, over his shoulders, up his back, and finally down to his naughty bits.

You could begin by lightly squeezing his joystick while giving him a light hand job. Once the allotted period of time has passed, you can then take further action, such as giving a firmer hand job or using your mouth to make him boil with delight and come. Wouldn't that be fantastic?

5. Give him a passionate kiss

Want to know a trick for making a man sob in bed? Hug him! And do it with fervor. One of the greatest pleasures he can enjoy before, during, and after making love is kissing.

But first, you must first prepare your lips. This entails using a quality lip balm to keep your lips soft and unquestionably free of chapping.

To avoid turning him off, make sure your breath is minty fresh and clean. You know, smell good because nobody wants to throw up.

Once you've finished, move on to a slow, one-time kiss with your partner, allowing it to last for a few seconds. After that, slowly pull your lips away from your partner's lips, keeping them close enough that they almost touch but do not (this lingering will heighten the passion and really grab your partner's full attention).

Then slant your head to the side and kiss him fervently. To ascertain pleasure, go slowly and deliberately.

You might want to try French kissing as the kiss develops, in which you gently insert your tongue into his mouth and allow it to dance with his tongue.

If you move your lips and use a small amount of tongue, kissing the jawline can also be enticing. Don't overlook your ears.

After that, slowly move your lips up his neck, chest, stomach, and finally to his groin. Grasp his joystick and encourage him with pleasure.

6. Role Play:Be Irresistible In Bed

Understanding your partner's fantasies can be crucial to learning how to make a man sob in bed. Whether he fantasizes about receiving a good spanking from a college professor, being taken advantage of by a doctor, or taking part in a gang bang, there is a way to satisfy all of his desires without him cheating, and this is where role-playing comes in.

By assuming different personas, acting out a scenario, and wooing or seducing your partner, you can increase his arousal through role playing. In order to fulfill his naughty fantasy, you assume a new identity in this romantic game.

Set the stage before you begin. A small physical change, such as donning a wig or changing your hairstyle from straight to curly or from brunette to blonde, can really help you get into the mindset of a new identity and help you lose yourself in the role.

And now that you have your outfit and your props, you can add some flair by going to a hotel bar and acting like two strangers who are going on their first date (just make sure you have reserved a room ahead of time).

Unable to afford that By changing the setting of your home, you can transform it into a hotel. For instance, you could transform your kitchen into an island or your dining room table into a makeshift bar for the evening, then start speaking with an accent from there if necessary.

Just let your partner know what is appropriate for him, and decide on a safe word that will stop the action the moment you feel uncomfortable.

7. Take the lead

Because they don't want to ruin their partner's perception of them as a "good girlfriend" or make him think they are strange, women are frequently reluctant to act inappropriately while they are in a committed relationship. Making your partner see your dominant, no-holds-barred side is one way to make him sob in bed.

This entails you exercising control over a submissive third party (your man) while engaging in these delightful acts of pleasure.

So take control for the evening and coerce your partner into bed. Ask him to take off those pants while gazing him in the face with those gorgeous eyes and telling him he can't talk, touch, or even move unless he is told to.

Do not even hesitate to ask him to go there. Alternating places occasionally would also let you assume control.

Get the upper hand and refuse to let him switch things up even if he tries so that you can maintain control. Since you have more control over the angle, speed, and depth from your position on top, be rough and unclean; bite, claw, scratch, spank, and pull his hair to seize the initiative.

He will tell you how he is feeling and whether he likes it, so don't ask. It's not your responsibility to please him; instead, focus on your own needs and demonstrate to him how you can have an absolute blast.

8. Moan For Your Man

We begin to lose control of our bodies when we are enjoying ourselves. The somatic nervous system is suppressed, and as a result, we are unable to control the sounds that emerge - ohh! Ooooooh! Ah! Ahh! Yeah!! Yes!!!

You can tell your partner he is doing a good job by moaning. It demonstrates how well he's pleasing you, which will encourage him to exert himself more while he's on you.

More often than not, it seems like you are reacting to his touches and letting him know how good you are feeling. That relieves a lot of pressure from him and boosts his ego because he can easily stimulate your erogenous zones.

So if you are a screamer, scream!!! Don't be reluctant. He doesn't want you to be forced to remain silent while hearing the creak of the bed.

While he grinds and thrusts you in time with your groans and screams of intense satisfaction, he wants to hear you whimper, growl, and scream his name. He awakens the beast inside of him the more you groan. That's how to make a man sob in bed, right there!

9. *Talk Dirty To A Man To Make Him Want You Bad*

You should also include dirty talking as you continue to think about how to make a man cry in bed. He wants to hear you whisper his ears the naughtiest ideas you've ever had.

So, if you were to say, "I want you to unzip my dress right now! " with a mischievous smile on your lips. It may cause some slight heating.

Get his mind and heart racing by going further to unleash the wild, romantic animal that isn't constrained by social conventions and rules in you: holy crap, I'm dripping wet, I need your c*ck! Take hold of my hair and treat me like your bitch. Keep going; it feels wonderful! You are overstuffed, etc.

This will enthuse him and keep things interesting in your relationship.

10. Examine various positions.

Variety is sometimes referred to as the "spice of life," and this is true. Stuck in a ruts can be monotonous and drive your man away. So, try assuming various positions to elicit his excitement.

Try the cowgirl or reverse style, corkscrew, the lotus, G-whiz, wheelbarrow, stand and deliver, etc. as alternatives to the standard missionary position.

He will like it when you feel tighter in some positions, and he may really like it when you can feel other parts of you more easily in other positions. Just have fun and come up with inventive things to do in bed.

11. Provide him with every visual

He might want this, but he won't ask for it. Men are visual creatures, and they would adore seeing that hot, bare body go above and beyond to make them feel fantastic.

So, when you're busy, be sure to give him the cold shoulder. Turn on the lights and let yourself be. You can take him to a mirror so that you can both see yourself performing (and/or add a camera for a better view later), and then let him see your face when you reach your climax.

This will leave him feeling eager and craving more, which is a surefire way to make a man want you badly.

12. Let Him Take Charge

He may occasionally try to take control of the situation by flipping you over, smacking your butt, (lightly) choking you, pinning your hands against the wall, tying you up, gripping your hair, and f**king you on the floor while your pants are being torn off or pulled to the side.

He wants to be in charge and have complete authority over you. Why don't you let him! Allow him to give you instructions on what to do to him and how to do it. Please comply with him as long as you don't get hurt (it's safe).

Any romantic relationship can be fueled by prioritizing intimacy and romantic gestures. How to keep husband happy at night will undoubtedly be achieved by kissing his lips, stroking his hair, and giving him a hard f-k.

Enjoy then!

CHAPTER 5 - Knowing Erogenous spots on men for great sex

Did you know that men have a spot on their bodies resembling a G-spot? It is known as the P-spot and is situated in the rectum, where the prostate can be accessed internally, in a region that is particularly sensitive to arousal and sexual stimulation.

For many men, this may not be news. What if I told you that this isn't the only body part that can produce these pleasurable sensations? Yes, it is accurate; therefore, pay close attention to what we have to say to you about them.

Pleasure points: what are they?

The pleasure points are areas of the body that, when stimulated, have a unique sexual awakening. Due to the abundance of nerve endings, certain body parts do tend to be more sensitive than others. We cannot ignore the physiological element, despite the fact that it exists. These pleasure points "activate or deactivate" depending on the state of our mind. In fact, many of these parts only become "awakened" when engaging in sex other than penetration.

So, do all men have the same erogenous zones? Can we group them? How can we get their attention? The solutions are here.

Erogenous zone types and stimulation techniques

Let's face it, there are some erogenous points that we are much more familiar with than others. Primary points, the most "popular," and secondary points, which are less extensively explored, are the two categories into which they are divided. The most "unexplored" ones will be left for the more daring ones later.

Primary points

The areas directly associated with sexual activity, such as the genitalia, are referred to as primary points and are typically shared by all men:

The penis is most likely a man's primary erogenous point. It is covered in nerve cells. The frenulum has the power to cause us to experience something particularly intense. You probably don't need any more proof that we can manipulate the penis however we please or that there are virtually endless ways to play with it.

Scrotum: the skin that protects the testicles. It should go without saying how delicate this region is, to the point where we can take advantage of it when it comes to sexual stimulation. Particularly enjoyable is the space between, known as the raphe. The caressing of this region with the tongue and lips can arouse many men. Due to the zone's sensitivity, it is necessary to experiment with the awakened sensations, which can range from tickling to pain.

Secondary points

These areas typically have a lot of potential to boost pleasure. Not every man will feel the same level of satisfaction. These issues are highly personal and individualized. In fact, some men experience orgasm through direct stimulation, despite the fact that these are not the "primary" points.

You can explore these erogenous areas alone or with a friend. But we have some suggestions for you to test out in a group to make your life easier. Tell your partner about these concepts if you want to discuss a particular angle.

One of the best-known and most amusing parts is the mouth and lips. Don't be afraid to experiment with different kisses. The texture and temperature of an ice cube can be explored in the mouth, stimulating the sense of touch. This is merely one of an infinite number of possibilities.

Touching or caressing the buttocks is a common weakness among men. Use your hands to make gentle movements in all directions. As soon as the sexual tension starts to rise, these movements will get more intense and pleasurable. Maybe now is the time to grab the buttocks firmly and with a passionate, desire-filled grip. Do you feel comfortable using your mouth on this private area of your body? That's receptiveness to novel experiences.

Nipples: This sensitive region has countless opportunities for stimulation. Having their lips or fingers caressed will greatly arouse some people. However, you might prefer to try light pinching and nibbling on the nipples if you prefer a more potent sensation.

Not just the nipples on the chest are erogenous points. Numerous exercises and methods can be used to stimulate the chest, which is a sizable area. Try to play with pressure and tension as you move from the upper part of the breast to the abdomen with kisses or caresses. Repeating this repeatedly results in a very strong arousal. Although if you try the same route with the tongue you can always add a plus...

Try to transition from complete relaxation to uncontrollable excitement at the nape of the neck. The issue is how. If this is new to you, it's best if your partner starts by gently kissing you between the Adam's apple and the collarbones. You could use your tongue if you're feeling particularly daring. What if you try using those bites we mentioned above if it's still not enough?

Ears: The earlobe is an especially delicate region. What you should avoid doing in this situation is arguably more interesting to know than what you can do. Avoid sticking your tongue in too far or blowing hard on the eardrum. The important thing is to treat this area of the body gently; the rest will come out naturally.

Additional erogenous areas

These might not be as well-known as the ones we've mentioned, but that doesn't make them any less thrilling. Undoubtedly, some of them will increase how much you enjoy your interactions:

Thighs: These are also a pleasurable body part, and as we approach the genital region, especially on the inner side, arousal rises. Try building up the sexual tension by moving from the lower area to the part that is closest to the genitals. Whatever method you choose to activate this zone is up to you.

When we use the term "navel," we primarily mean the region between the navel and the genitalia. When stimulated, this abdominal path can lead to an increase in sexual tension. This is the "continuation" of the chest proposal, if you have already read it. Due to the blood flow in this area, there is a lot of sexual tension when we move our lips over it. Don't forget the hip bones, as the sensations won't make you forget them.

Back: is a roomy enough space to let our fantasies about certain sexual encounters run wild. Ice was already mentioned as a potential addition, but what about erotic candles? The back's sensitivity makes it especially ideal to begin experimenting with temperature contrasts that will elicit a wide range of sensations.

Yes, the palm, the back, and the fingers of the hands can excite someone. You can use feathers, various textiles (such as silk), or your lips and tongue to arouse new sensations.

Eyelids: Because so many nerves converge here, this area of the body is extremely sensitive. With our eyes closed, gentle kisses and circular caresses can stimulate this area.

Knees: In reality, the part of the body that can tickle the most is the back (hamstring). It all depends on how it is stimulated: with hands, lips, or tongue. Play with different pressures.

Armpits: Especially the lower portion near the chest, the armpits have a lot of erotic potential. The folds and curves have a unique sensitivity. This area has a very high potential for excitement. Once more, eroticism is the ability to arouse a pleasurable sensation in a body part that can tickle us.

The "Prohibited" zones

There are obviously no off-limits areas on the human body. However, given their location and the stigma they carry—they have been associated with taboos and stigmas since ancient times—the erogenous points that we will discuss below are particularly contentious. Nevertheless, we recognize that it is time to eliminate and get rid of them. This is why:

The perineum, or "L-spot," The area of the body that runs from the scrotum to the anus is known as the superficial side of the pubococcygeus muscle. It is called the L-spot because when it is stimulated, its nerve endings can provide us with a great deal of pleasure. Since it externally stimulates the male prostate, it is actually a region that is closely related to ejaculation and the intensity experienced during an orgasm. Compared to the arousal we experience with the penis, this stimulation produces a more progressive response that also reaches "deeper" intensities.

If you're just starting out, try massaging in circular motions with your middle and index fingers. You control the massage's level of vigor. Depending on how we are feeling, we can go farther (or less).

Anus (P-spot): Even the outermost portion of the anal walls is extremely sensitive. Therefore, stimulating this region is one way to boost libido. Do not be afraid to give it a try; if done with proper hygiene precautions, it is a safe and very possibly enjoyable practice. even to say again.

The well-known P-spot, which is housed inside the anus, enters the picture at this point. On its anterior side, this location has a connection to the prostate nerves. To access it, one must insert a finger, for instance, and apply light pressure to this wall in the shape of a hook. After that, you can make gentle pressures and movements, though it's normal to experience some discomfort the first time. Never be afraid to take your time.

On the other hand, it's crucial to remember that activating the P-spot has advantages for sexual satisfaction in addition to reducing the risk of prostate cancer. Studies have shown that activating the P-spot is a reliable method of stopping this specific form of cancer.

What if the erogenous zones were combined? These spots have an unexplainable ability to awaken sensations. By massaging the earlobes while stroking the nipples, for example, we can stimulate more than one of these points simultaneously.

Try both masturbating and stimulating the P-spot at the same time. When you first begin using anal touch, when you are not yet accustomed to its sensations, this can be especially helpful.

The value of stimulating touch

The crucial "zones" of pleasure are there, but you already know where they are and how to activate them. We do not want you to undervalue the value of affectionate touch, though.

It's crucial to keep in mind that there are different kinds of stimulation. As a result, giving and receiving kisses is a sign of love, intimacy, support, and, of course, eroticism.

Caresses should be integrated into sexual encounters in order to explore and discover our preferences and constraints as well as to set difficulties like what unique practices might be tried. Through caresses, discovering these horizons takes on a completely new experience.

What physical element is usually present from beginning to end? Touching each other during sexual encounters is a typical part of the entire erotic process in the majority of couples. They serve as both the climax of desire and the final wave of goodbye most of the time. Given this, expressing and receiving affection is just as significant as sexual arousal.

Conclusion

The treasures of real eroticism are hidden within our body, which is a fantastic map. We can either look for them alone or with other people, which is good news. Although some of the places we've listed are satisfying in and of themselves, others might make us feel unwelcome, and still others will compel us to go back repeatedly.

Maybe it's also time to add some playfulness to your routines, or even some pain, though we'll talk more about that in a later article. In other words, the possibilities are endless. Always remember that you are the one who sets the limits!

CHAPTER 6 - Giving him a good blowjob

Your grade for this assignment is going to be an A+.

The mighty blow job is undoubtedly intimidating, but it's also probably one of the best sex acts you can perform for pleasure. Even though having complete control over your partner's strap-on or penis can feel empowering, you might occasionally consider refining your blow job technique. After all, how exactly do you perform a good blow? No doubt, sex education didn't address this.

It really depends on personal preferences, though. However, getting a blow job alone is a huge turn on for many people. In addition, a lot of people get excited by the visual aspect of watching their penis slide in and out of a mouth. Not to mention that no one can replicate the sensation of a blow job on their own, unlike a hand job or even penetrative sex (obviously). Your lips and tongue are living, moving, priceless works of art, but your mouth is wet and warm like a vagina (or a lubed-up hand).

Although it's not for everyone, a blow job can be a great way to increase affection when you and your partner are really clicking.

So returning to technique, what additional information should you have about blow jobs beyond the uh, fundamentals? So, if you want to up your oral sex game, this is exactly how to do it.

1. Show enthusiasm.

The most important guideline for giving good head is to genuinely want to give good head.

This is not to say that you should act as though you enjoy doing something in the bedroom if you don't. (In that vein, never comply with a sexual partner's request simply because it makes you uncomfortable.) However, the best thing you can bring to the BJ party is a positive attitude if you're thinking about going down on someone, which, if you're reading this, it seems like you are.

Here are a few techniques for expressing your enthusiasm:

Establish eye contact. Avoid staring at someone for an extended period of time without blinking (creepy), but do take deliberate breaks to shift your focus from their penis to their eyes while observing all facial cues. (You sexpot, this is also a great opportunity to bat your lashes and "smize"!)

Inform them of your heightened arousal. You know how when a partner puts you down, you can feel self-conscious? Yes, everyone can! So congratulate yourself on how excited you are as a result of how difficult they are to swallow. Or just say it out loud: "I adore the sensation of your penis in my mouth." Simple but powerful.

Inquire about their desires. By requesting feedback, you demonstrate your concern and desire to provide your partner with the best experience possible. Just before placing your mouth back on the shaft, you can ask "How does this feel?" or halfway through, "Is this wet enough for you?" One thing to avoid asking is, "Hello, are you close yet?" Make it simple if your partner isn't comfortable answering questions during a blowout: Have them hold your hand and squeeze it whenever they feel good. It will be simpler for you to determine which moves they really enjoy, and it will give you a nice confidence boost throughout.

2. Add your hands to the action.

Although a blow job may qualify as oral sex, your mouth is not required to perform all the necessary tasks.

After a few minutes of work, if your jaw begins to hurt or feel fatigued, you're probably sucking with your mouth too forcefully. As a result, transfer some of the work to your hands and rely on their pressure.

Once you've warmed up a little, try this basic stroke:

Add your mouth after wrapping your dominant hand around the shaft.

Connect your hand to your lips by sealing them there with your thumb and index finger (which are forming the letter "O").

Your hand and lips should be moved up and down the penis.

You can keep your mouth closed and move your wet hand up and down separately if their penis is larger than average.

After that, you can experiment a little with your hand technique.

Wrist Twist: Try it out. Move your hand up and down while rotating your firm wrist in clockwise circles with your mouth on the penis (this is still oral sex).

Once you've established your position, use your other hand to participate in the game. Focus on more than just your penis, advises Anderson. Some people prefer having their leg touched while having their nipples stimulated, making the experience more sensory-rich overall. whenever possible Squeeze the balls gently in the cup.

3. Do not be hesitant to include spit (lots of it).

Although everyone has their own, er, preferred levels of moisture, I've discovered that most people concur that a good blow job requires a lot of saliva. Whenever the penis begins to feel a little dry, try to do some **sexy** spitting (read: make it subtle) without going overboard to the point where your hand starts to slide all over the place.

In light of this, it wouldn't hurt to keep a glass of water handy to prevent dry mouth—you never know when you might need it.

4. Try to keep your tongue as loose and soft as possible.

Your tongue gives a blow job the warmth, the texture, and the dampness that they can't get from anywhere else.

When you're moving up and down (which is most of your job), keep your tongue soft in your mouth, and then use the tip of your tongue to trace the head and frenulum—the underside where the penis head (if circumcised) meets the shaft.

Expect your partner to lose it in those two areas, especially the frenulum, which is dense with nerve endings.

Additionally, you can perform a few tongue flicks or lick from the very bottom of the shaft to the very tip and back down again.

5. Pretend to say the word "purple" as you are about to.

Try to maintain a fish-faced smile while sucking; pretend to be about to say "purple." Your lips automatically contort into the ideal head-giving pout when you say that word; they are slightly pillowy and curled, which makes them feel wetter and creates the ideal suction.

Thank you very much.

6. Modify the visual.

The visual aspect of a blow job is very important. You can also experiment with positioning yourself in various areas of the space, such as having your partner stand up against the wall and you kneel in front of them. You can even stand in front of a mirror so they can see you from all sides.

7. If you enjoy the deep throat, try it.

Deep throating, where the member is taken into the throat, is unquestionably an advanced technique. Why? Gag reflex, two words.

Some people's gag reflexes are easier to trigger than others, but if you can train yours, you can shock (and I mean SHOCK) your partner occasionally with deep throat clearing.

Their mouth is obviously smaller than yours, so deepthroating feels amazing to them. It's also seductive to see their entire length fit inside your mouth. (Going back to the previous point's visual.)

Warning: Start slowly and only when you can breathe comfortably through your nose. There is no penis worth choking on.

8. Lie down and relax.

Nothing is worse than giving a blow job while experiencing knee or neck pain from an awkward or unsupportive position. In order to make the situation more enjoyable for everyone involved, make sure you (and your partner) are in comfortable positions. A fun way to experiment and reduce pressure and stress is to try out various positions. Both parties will be able to tell pretty quickly if one position isn't working, so have fun with it and try something else! This increases the overall enjoyment of the process.

9. Moisten it.

Lube is crucial. And it completely alters all forms of sexual activity. Although saliva production can be challenging, especially if you're thirsty or stay in a dry environment, moisture is undoubtedly a key component of blow jobs. For both parties, having a dry mouth is unpleasant. To increase wettability and pleasure, add some lube.

There are many lube options to choose from that can change your blow job game, whether you like the taste of coconut oil or prefer an oral lube.

10. Determine your ideal outcome.

Knowing what you want or need at the time of ejaculation is essential if you want to be a giver. Okay, if swallowing and ejaculating in your mouth don't cause any major problems. If it is, however, you must notify everyone in advance of any workarounds.

It's up to you how you handle the ejaculation portion of a blow job. If you prefer not to ejaculate through your mouth, ask your partner to signal when the time is right. Then, shut your mouth and ejaculate instead with your hand. They can also spit it out if they don't mind the cum but don't want to swallow it.

11. Cover those canines.

Blowjobs and teeth don't really go together. But since teeth make up a sizable portion of mouths, understanding how to handle them during a blow job is crucial. Your ability to move up and down the shaft is aided by a tongue that is loosely covering your teeth. Another suggestion is to slightly wrap your lips around your teeth to prevent canine contact.

12. Think about giving an ice cream cone a lick.

Consider how you would lick an ice cream cone as a technique. Move your tongue and mouth along the shaft slowly. Build up to actually putting it in your mouth completely; the anticipation will drive them crazy.

13. Experiment with temperature

Bring the ice and the heat. Yes, it is definitely very enticing to use ice cubes during a blow job. This unusual technique may sound like a blow job urban legend, but stuffing crushed ice into your mouth causes a tingling sensation that can be reviving due to the contrast between your warm mouth and the cool ice.

Play with ice with your partner's permission. Try taking a sip from an ice cube just before you slam into them. Go to town by putting crushed ice in your mouth. Although the combination of the cold and melting ice may make you feel like a chipmunk, it makes for a wet, enjoyable time. Trust me, give it a shot.

14. *Think about condoms.*

Nobody considers using a condom for a blowout, but they can prevent STDs! And it's crucial to engage in safe sexual behavior. It's a good thing there are flavored condoms and lube to make it more enjoyable.

15. *Feel it out*

Spend some time using your mouth to explore. Each penis is unique. Use your mouth to feel the texture, shape, and mouth-filling quality of the object. Investigate it with interest.

Unless that's your thing, in which case more power to ya, you don't have to jump into a blow job and go straight for the deep throat. Instead of clenching, consider how your mouth might be used to seal a tighter envelope around this penis.

Recall: Release the pressure of performing an orgasm. If you're overly concerned with getting that, it might even ruin your enjoyment. Instead, the key to pleasing your partner is to concentrate on the journey of pleasure, both in receiving and giving.

How can I tell if I did a good blowjob?

There is no objective way to know if you did a good job because it depends entirely on what your partner likes and what the intended outcome is. The ability to make your partner cum is not the only indicator of a good blow job; you can perform a superb blow job even if the goal is merely to increase arousal or induce orgasm. If the body experiences pleasure and displays contentment, you can be confident that you're acting appropriately.

It's crucial to understand that orgasm and ejaculation are not indicators of a successful blow job. Typically, the recipient of the blow job will say, "Oh wow that was amazing." They probably would have asked you to stop during it if it weren't good.

Giving a good blow job also requires good communication before, after, and during. A crucial aspect of emotional vulnerability that only supports your sex life is talking about it both during and after.

Open-ended questions, such as "What did you like about that?" or "What was your favorite part?" should be posed to your partner. The question "If we could do something differently next time, what would that be?" or "What's one thing you really want me to make sure I include next time that you really like?" are two more that might be appropriate.

CHAPTER 7 - Sex positions that all men adore

Many men believe that there are many wonderful aspects of sex. After all, it's a ton of fun and feels fantastic. However, there are some characteristics of some positions that make them even more advantageous for men than other positions.

Missionary

This traditional sex position has nothing not to be adored. Men adore it, despite the fact that it might not seem to have some of the advantages of other sex positions. It enables them to take control of the pace, kiss you, and place their face in the nape of your neck while doing so. They can also reach out and touch and kiss your breasts.

Female at top

When you are the best missionary, men adore you. They are allowed to kiss your mouth, neck, and breasts. You can also look each other in the eye. Men enjoy watching you in this position because they have no control over the pace and can see you in all of your sexy, hot glory. They can also easily grab your buttocks while you are doing this while on top of them.

Doggy style

Doggy style is yet another sex position that men adore to the hilt. He is not only getting deeper when he hits it from behind, but he is also able to grab onto your hips because he can see your buttocks wiggle. It feels primal to him, which is another benefit for him.

Cowgirl

Men adore this particular sex position very much. They get to put their hands wherever they want, have their woman do all the work, and can see everything—including your bouncing breasts. Men adore it as well for the incredible feeling it gives them while taking in the magnificent view.

Reverse cowgirl

Similar to why they adore cowgirls, men adore this. They see an amazing view of your back and buttocks this time. They can feel up your buttocks and hips and can delve deeper because their woman is doing the work.

69

Men adore being in this position because it makes them happy to please their women. Both do the work and leave at the same time, rather than one person doing all the work and satisfying everyone involved. Because of the view, men also adore this position.

He bends, and you sit.

The woman then kneels on top of the man as he sits. Men adore this position because it allows them to hold you close and have a very intimate interaction with you. Men also enjoy this because they can ride you while kissing your lips, neck, or even your breasts.

Hovering butterfly

Men adore this position because their partner is seated on their face while they are giving oral in the most comfortable position. Men adore being able to taste and feel everything underground. They also enjoy being able to grab onto your buttocks, stomach, hips, and breasts.

www.ingramcontent.com/pod-product-compliance
Lightning Source LLC
Chambersburg PA
CBHW061616250726
48653CB00019B/1988